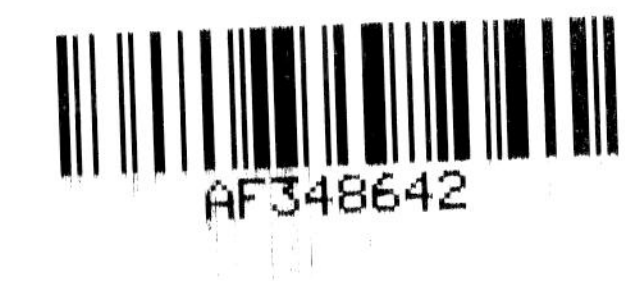
AF348642

Made in the USA
Monee, IL
07 July 2026

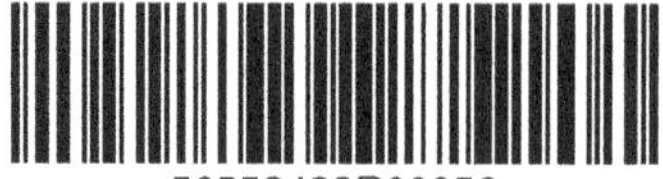

56552433R00056